T0296181

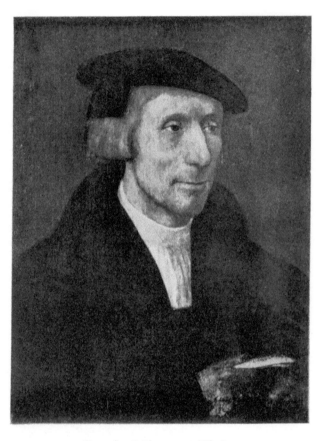

THOMAS LINACRE

Portrait of Linacre at Windsor

Linacre Lecture, 1908
St John's College, Cambridge

THOMAS LINACRE

by

WILLIAM OSLER, M.D., F.R.S.

REGIUS PROFESSOR OF MEDICINE IN THE
UNIVERSITY OF OXFORD

CAMBRIDGE:
at the University Press
1908

CAMBRIDGE
UNIVERSITY PRESS

University Printing House, Cambridge CB2 8BS, United Kingdom

Published in the United States of America by Cambridge University Press, New York

Cambridge University Press is part of the University of Cambridge.

It furthers the University's mission by disseminating knowledge in the pursuit of
education, learning and research at the highest international levels of excellence.

www.cambridge.org
Information on this title: www.cambridge.org/9781107425750

© Cambridge University Press 1908

First published 1908
First paperback edition 2014

A catalogue record for this publication is available from the British Library

ISBN 978-1-107-42575-0 Paperback

CONTENTS

PLATES

CONTENTS

PLATES

I

INTRODUCTION AND LIFE

Bound by the invisible links of common interests, the social and educational points of contact between the old Universities only serve to bring into sharp relief their complementary contrasts. Rivals now-a-days less in the prowess of brains than of brawn, throughout the centuries there has never lacked in each a keen appreciation of the merits and defects of the other. However much a modern Thomas Caius may boast of the superiority of Oxford, with his great namesake John he feels in his heart that things are better managed here; and it is well known in the combination rooms that when he speaks of Oxford the tongue of a

Cambridge man is very apt to belie his heart. Migrations from one place to the other have gone on for centuries; incorporations, less frequent now than formerly, have counteracted to some extent the ill effects of close breeding. Oxford men have adorned Cambridge chairs, and as Oxford Professors Cambridge men have solved the riddle of dual personality. And the Universities are linked in the possession of the blessed memory of a group of men whose benefactions make them honoured as much in the one as in the other. Among those in order the first, and in scholarship the most distinguished stands Thomas Linacre. A summary of his life and character is thus given in the epitaph placed by Caius on a stately monument in old St Pauls surmounted by a phoenix[1];

---

[1] Apropos of the phoenix Fuller could not resist one of his characteristic remarks, "Yea, I may call these doctors the two Phoenixes of their profession in our nation and justify the expression, seeing the latter in some sort sprang from the ashes of the former."

" Thomas Lynacrus, Regis Henrici VIII medicus ; vir Graece et Latine atque in re medica longe eruditissimus : Multos aetate sua languentes, et qui jam animam desponderant, vitae restituit; Multa Galeni opera in Latinam linguam, mira et singulari facundia vertit: Egregium opus de emendata structura Latini sermonis, amicorum rogatu, paulo ante mortem edidit. Medicinae studiosis Oxoniae publicas lectiones duas, Cantabrigiae unam, in perpetuum stabilivit. In hac urbe Collegium Medicorum fieri sua industria curavit, cujus et Praesidens proximus electus est. Fraudes dolosque mire perosus ; fidus amicis ; omnibus ordinibus juxta clarus; aliquot annos antequam obierat Presbyter factus ; plenus annis, ex hac vita migravit, multum desideratus, Anno Domini 1524, die 20 Octobris. Vivit post Funera virtus."

Nearly four centuries have now passed since the endowment of his lectureships at

Oxford and Cambridge. Vacant, by the happy translation of Dr Donald MacAlister to the Principalship of Glasgow University, this College, as guardian of the trust, has decided to change the lectureship to an annual lecture to be called after the name of the founder. That you, Master and Fellows of St John's College, should have asked one from Linacre's University to give this first lecture manifests in the sons of the prophets the old courtesy of the fathers. In the choice of a subject you will all agree that on the occasion of such a radical change a review of the life and works of the Founder is most appropriate, and here duty and inclination meet, since it happens that for some years I have been interested in both.

What we know of the early years of Linacre may be told in the brief sentences of Freind, "Canterbury gave him his birth (1460) and

Oxford his education; he was chosen in 1484 Fellow of All Souls[1]." His college is not known, nor have we a single item of information about his studies or his mode of life. Whether or not he was a kinsman of the Founder of All Souls is disputed. At Canterbury he had come under the care of William de Selling, possibly a relative, a man already infected with the new learning, and while an undergraduate Grocyn and Latimer became his friends and the names remain as the Oxford triumvirate with whom true English scholarship begins. Studies scholastic, life monastic express in a sentence Oxford at the end of the 15th century. Wood describes the condition in a paragraph: "The schools were much frequented with quirks and sophistry. All things, whether taught or written, seemed to be trite and inane. No pleasant streams of humanity or mythology were gliding among us;

[1] *History of Physic*, Vol. II.

and the Greek language, from whence the greater part of knowledge is derived, was at a very low ebb or in a manner forgotten." That good son of the church and of the profession, Dr James J. Walsh, has recently published a charming book on *The Thirteenth, the greatest of the Centuries*, and he makes a very good case for what is sometimes called the first Renaissance. Had the times been ripe and could men have done it, such men as Roger Bacon and Robert of Lincoln and Richard de Bury would have made, for England at least, a new birth ; but from an intellectual standpoint the 13th century was at best, not the true dawn brightening more and more unto the perfect day, but a glorious Aurora, which flickered down again into the arctic night of mediaevalism.

Not until Greece rose from the dead did light and liberty come to the human mind, and it is the special glory of Linacre that he became, as Fuller says, the "restorer of learning in this country." But certain manuscript treasures in the Bodleian and in the libraries of Balliol, New and Lincoln Colleges, Oxford, tell of an intermediate though unsuccessful Oxford movement by a group of men remembered now only by a few who know their story. An English medical student, one John Free, a Balliol man, became not only the most learned Englishman of his age, but was the first who ever attempted the goal of universal learning Italy had created. A peripatetic professor of medicine in the North Italian Universities, he was the prototype of the English scholars, who for the next two hundred years were to flock across the Alps as "o'er a brook." But Free, Grey, Flemming, Gunthrop and Tiptoft, all Oxonians and all, save Flemming, Balliol men, had no enduring influence on English scholarship, and the manuscript treasures collected in Italy and now

distributed in the Oxford libraries alone remain
to tell of this abortive renaissance.

William de Selling, Linacre's teacher, had
already been in Italy and had studied Greek
and had brought back manuscripts to Canterbury, of the monastery of which he became
Prior. It is stated that the first real facilities to
learn in England were there to be found, and
he translated from the Greek a work of St John
Chrysostom. It is not improbable that Linacre
went to Oxford knowing Greek, and already
athirst for the new learning. In 1488 Selling
was sent by Henry VII on an embassy to the
Pope, and we can imagine how eagerly the
young Oxford scholar grasped the opportunity
to visit Italy with his teacher. According to
Leland, Linacre was to have taken part in the
embassy to Rome, but at Bologna, meeting
his old teacher Poliziano and naturally thinking
the advantages too great to be neglected,

de Selling left Linacre with him[1]. How long he stayed is uncertain. We hear of him next at Florence still under the tutorship of Poliziano at the Court of Lorenzo the Magnificent. Here he seems to have had the advantages of sharing in the instruction given to the young princes, Piero and Giovanni. Years afterwards to the younger brother, when Pope Leo X, Linacre dedicated one of his works. In addition to the instruction of Poliziano he came under the influence of the great Greek scholar, Demetrius Chalcondyles. What a contrast for the young All-Souls' Fellow to exchange the dreary semi-monastic life for the polished world at the Court of Lorenzo where he associated with the master spirits of the age. He may have sat at the same board with Michael Angelo, with Marsilio Ficino and with Pico

[1] Dr Sandys tells me that there is no ground for believing that Linacre met Politian at Bologna.

della Mirandola. We do not know what the
austere young Oxonian thought of the frivolities
and diversions of Lorenzo and his companions;
possibly he joined in them, but however much
he may have appreciated the learning of
Poliziano he did not make that genial heathen
his life model. After a stay of a year or more
he went to Rome, where he came under the
influence of another great scholar, Hermolaus
Barbarus. Johnson quotes the following anec-
dote of their accidental meeting: "He was one
day engaged in the Vatican, in an examination
of the Phaedon of Plato, when Hermolaus
Barbarus suddenly approached the press where
he was seated, and expressed his conviction
that the stranger had no claim, like himself, to
the epithet Barbarus, from his choice of the
book to which his attention was directed.
Linacre recognised the speaker, notwithstanding
the equivocation under which his name was

communicated; and this accidental interview became the foundation of a firm and lasting friendship, which was afterwards improved by the similarity of their dispositions and pursuits."

Though not a physician, Barbarus was at this time intensely interested in the works of Dioscorides, preparing his well-known edition, and possibly from him Linacre may have received the impulse to study medicine. From him too, most likely, came that accurate and critical knowledge of Aristotle, for which Linacre became famous among his friends. Barbarus has left a charming account of his literary life, ideal in every respect, and one can imagine the zeal with which under the direction of such a man Linacre examined and collated some of the priceless manuscripts of the Vatican. It must have been at this period that he had access to the Greek manuscripts of Galen's works from which he made the translations published many years after. He is mentioned, indeed, by one writer among the Calligraphi or transcribers of early Greek manuscripts. Johnson draws a parallel between the lives of Barbarus and of Linacre, particularly in their love of letters and of retirement, their celibate life and in their indifference to honours. We next hear of Linacre at Venice, the friend and companion of the great scholar and printer, Aldus, whose editions of the classics remain unrivalled monuments of his art and of his erudition. They seem to have become fast friends, and Aldus employed him in literary work, and he edited and translated Proclus *on the Sphere*, published in 1499. In the dedication of the work to the Prince of Carpi, Aldus pays a high tribute to the scholarship of Linacre. Payne points out the very interesting fact that in the Aldine *Editio princeps* of Aristotle there is an allusion to Linacre indicating that he had something to do with the editing or correcting of that great work. Linacre's own private copy, a superb edition on vellum, with his autograph, is one of the treasures of the library at New College. From the dates at which these volumes were issued, 1495—1497, it is quite possible Linacre may have been at the time resident in Venice.

After Free, Linacre was one of the earliest of the English students to seek a medical education at Padua then and after one of the most famous schools in Europe. We do not know how long he remained or who were his teachers, but he is stated to have taken the doctor's degree with more than usual applause. There is no warrant for the statement sometimes made that he became a professor. In connection with Linacre's subsequent work as a grammarian, an interesting Paduan incident is referred to by Richard Pacey, Ambassador from Henry VIII to the State of Venice. Grammar and Rhetoric dispute as to the mutual excellencies of Theodorus Gaza and Linacre: "Grammar first claims Linacre as her own, Rhetoric contends that he was by right her son, and that Grammar was only the occupation of his leisure moments. On one occasion (says Rhetoric) he condescended to dispute with some Grammarian on certain minutiae connected with the vocative case, but gained a more brilliant victory when he defended his theses for graduation at Padua." Even at that date the North Italian medical schools were very highly organized. It is a revelation to read in Ferrari's monograph[1] of the long list of teachers at Pavia in the middle of the 15th century. Johnson states that Linacre's route from Padua may be accurately and precisely traced. "Pursuing his course through Vicenza, Verona,

[1] Une Chaire de Médecine au XVe Siècle, Paris, 1899.

Brescia, Bergamo and Milan, he crossed the Rhone and rested a short time in the Pays de Cevennes, a mountainous and romantic district of France, extending from the source of the Loire to the north of Languedoc, and occupying the tract of country between the ancient Aquitania and Gallia Narbonensis. Here he indulged in the ceremony of erecting an altar on the summit of the highest mountain of Cevennes, and of dedicating it to the country, which he had just left, as the parent of his studies and of his literary application"—Sancta Mater Studiorum. We do not know where Johnson got his authority for these statements or where he found the poems which he published in which two friends lament Linacre's departure from Italy. Of one visit we know, namely, to the celebrated Nicolaus Leonicenus, of Vicenza, one of the earliest and most distinguished of the medical humanists and author of the first treatise on Syphilis, at this time beginning to rage in Europe. He may have remained with him for some time, as Leonicenus speaks of Linacre as his pupil (Payne). In any case he must have found in the old Ferrara professor a remarkable character. He read the physic lectures for upwards of seventy years[1].

The length of Linacre's stay in Italy is not certain. Johnson says two years, but Payne thinks the evidence is in favour of a longer residence, six or seven years. Returning to England Linacre resumed his work at Oxford, teaching Greek, and probably practising medicine. Little is known of his life at this period. He had as friends the great scholars, Grocyn,

[1] In answer to one who asked him why he did not practise his art Leonicenus replied that he did the public a greater service by teaching those who cured them. He held that Philosophy and *belles lettres* should be joined to medicine, and when at the age of 96 he was asked to what he attributed his great age, he replied, to the innocency of his customs, the tranquillity of his soul and the frugality of his diet.

Latimer and Colet, all, like himself, deeply in-terested in promoting the new learning. More was his pupil, and Erasmus, who at this time came to Oxford to study Greek with him, became a life-long friend. There are in the letters of Erasmus many references to his teachers of this period. One is the well known and oft quoted, " In Colet I hear Plato himself. Who does not admire the perfect compass of science in Grocyn? What can be more acute, more profound or more refined than the judge-ment of Linacre?" We cannot but regret that Erasmus did not leave on record a character sketch of Linacre similar to those unrivalled descriptions in which he has immortalised More and Colet. To this group of remarkable men England owed the introduction of the new learning. At the instigation of and under the direction of Barbarus the three friends, Linacre, Grocyn and Latimer, undertook the

translation into Latin of the works of Aristotle,
and it is said that Linacre completed his part.
Erasmus refers to his version of the meteorolo-
gical works in flattering terms, but the work
never appeared. Meanwhile Linacre's reputation as a scholar and physician was increasing,
but about 1500 the peaceful academic life was
interrupted by a call to court as tutor to Prince
Arthur.

Possibly he may have had an earlier connection with this prince, as to him he dedicates his
first work, Proclus *de Sphera*. As this book
stands somewhat apart from his others, I may
refer to it here quite briefly. It was published from the Aldine Press in 1499 and
appears in a thick folio containing a large
number of old Astronomical works—*Astronomici
Veteres.* The original Greek is published with
the Latin translation. This became a very
popular work and was reprinted very frequently.

There are 14 editions in the British Museum.
Aldus regrets that Linacre has not sent him his
edition of Simplicius on Aristotle's Physics and
on Aristotle's *Meteora* that they might have
accompanied the shorter work. And then he
inserts a letter from Grocyn in which the older
scholar thanks the great publisher for his kind
treatment of Linacre. This has a special interest
as the only known piece of writing (except his
well-known snow-ball epigram) of the great
scholar whose reputation as a Grecian was
unrivalled in England.

Early in the century Linacre became the
King's physician, and Erasmus mentions him as
one of the special adornments of a court "less a
palace than an academy of learning." At that
period, indeed for many years later, there was a
very close affiliation between the medical and
the clerical profession. It was not an uncommon
thing for a learned divine to practise physic, and

on the other hand a considerable number of distinguished physicians, among whom may be mentioned Marsilius Ficinus and John Clement, became priests. Linacre, too, joined this group of φιλοθεολογιατρόνομοι as it has been called. The date of his ordination is not known, but about the year 1509 he began to receive preferment in the church and he became in succession Rector of Mersham in Kent, Prebend of Wells, Incumbent of Hawkhurst, Canon and prebend of the Collegiate Chapel of St Stephen, Westminster, Prebend of York, Rector of Holworthy, and Rector of Wigan. Many of these livings he resigned shortly after receiving and it is quite probable that the sale was a source of profit, as was so common in those days when the evils of pluralism were not regarded very seriously. From a statement made to his friend, the Archbishop of Canterbury, he seemed to have taken orders with the view to obtain the necessary leisure for his literary work. Busy with this and still in practice, and with the organization of the great foundation in London and the benefactions to the two Universities, his life must have been one of great activity. As age came he began to suffer with stone in the bladder, to which he finally succumbed on the 20th of October, 1524.

II

MEDICAL HUMANIST

Linacre did more than take an active share in the revival of learning in England. Upon us of his profession he has a very special claim as one of the most distinguished of the medical humanists—that interesting band of 15th and 16th century scholars who sought to break Arabian domination and to restore to medicine the uncorrupted spirit of Greece. During the scholastic period the knowledge of Greek medicine had filtered in a very imperfect and defective form through the great Arabian writers who absolutely controlled medical thought. The authors of the 13th, 14th and 15th centuries were little more than commentators on the Arabians. Thus in a popular text-book, the *Practica* of Ferrari (1472), it is stated that there are 3,110 references to Avicenna, 1280 to Rhazes, and 1160 to Galen, 540 to Mesué. In the interesting catalogue of the library of this author a very large proportion of the books were commentaries on Arabian authors. A revolt against this domination spread widely throughout the North Italian Universities, and everywhere men became filled with a burning desire to purify the polluted doctrines of the Fathers. But the devotion was by no means confined to Hippocrates and Galen. It was in no narrow spirit that these men went to work. As we have seen, Linacre had undertaken with his friends, Grocyn and Latimer, a translation of Aristotle, and we have the authority of Erasmus that Linacre had finished his section. Plato, too, came within the sphere of their devotion, and the well-known Lyons physician, Champier, published a little book, *Symphonia Platonis*, (Plate III) etc., in which the frontispiece shows an orchestra composed of Hippocrates, Plato, Aristotle, and Galen, the four princes of medicine executing a symphony with their violins. As I have mentioned in another place[1], among the men of the latter 15th and early 16th centuries, given in chronological order in Bayle's *Biographie Medicale*, more than one half had translated or edited works of Galen and Hippocrates. In reality it was not so much that they swept away the impurities in Arabian

[1] Harveian Oration, 1907.

medicine as that they restored to the profession Greek ideals, and again made observation and experiment the Alpha and Omega of the science. During his stay in Italy, Linacre had had many opportunities to consult the manuscripts of Galen, many of which he collated and transcribed. It seems to have been well known among his friends that he was at work upon these translations and it was only at their urgent solicitation that they were printed. The first one to appear was Galen's *de Sanitate Tuenda*, Paris (Rubens), 1517, a handsome folio with wide margins and very good type (Plate IV). The work was dedicated to Henry VIII. In the British Museum there is a beautiful copy on vellum with an illuminated title page and initial letters and a manuscript dedicated to Cardinal Wolsey. This was a very popular book, frequently reprinted, of which there are five editions in the British Museum.

The second was a larger work, the *Methodus Medendi*, a fine folio also published in Paris by Matheu, 1519 (Plate V). It too was dedicated to Henry VIII. In the preface Linacre refers to two previous books, and both Johnson and Payne mention this as difficult to explain since, so far as we know, only the *de Sanitate Tuenda* had been previously published. The explanation is given by Mr Joseph Manning[1] who points out that Claudius Chevalonius, who lived at the Sign of the Golden Sun, Paris, in a petition to his readers before his edition of the *Methodus Medendi* says—that these twenty books, meaning the *de Sanitate Tuenda* containing six books, and the *Methodus Medendi* fourteen, embrace the three principal parts of medicine, and he adds "Candid reader, whoever thou art that hast drawn profit from them pray well for Linacre the Englishman who has translated them with the

[1] *Notes and Queries*, Series VIII, Vol. IV.

utmost possible fidelity." Hieronymus Mercu-
rialis also refers to the three parts of medicine
—therapeutics, hygiene and gymnastics—corres-
ponding to Aristotle's goods of the body, health,
strength and beauty. The *Methodus Medendi*
became a very popular book and was frequently
reprinted. The British Museum has a 1526
and 1538 edition.

The third of his translations *de Temperamentis* (Plate VI) has a special interest here
as it comes from an early Cambridge press,
and is one of the first books issued in
England in which Greek types were used and
the first book with a copper-plate title. It
was published by Siberch in 1521 in small
quarto. There is in the Bodleian a very
fine copy printed on vellum which was given
to the Library by my distinguished pre-
decessor, Sir Thomas Clayton, in the 17th
century.

Two years later a fourth work of Galen was published by Pynson in 1523, *de Naturalibus Facultatibus* (Plate VII). The fifth work, Galen's short tract, *de Pulsuum Usu* (Plate VIII), was published by Pynson about the same time, though no date is given. The sixth work, *de Symptomatum Differentiis*, was published by Pynson in 1524 just after Linacre's death. These translations at once became popular, particularly on the continent where they were reprinted separately, and they very soon began to appear in the collected editions of Galen. As early as 1528 they all appeared in a Lyons collection edited by Rivierus, dedicated to one of the sons of his friend, Champier—twenty-three of Galen's works translated by Valla, Leonicenus, Copus, Laurentianus, &c. Underneath is the quaint legend which indicates the depth of feeling at the time—*Hi sunt qui e Barbarorum faucibus Galenum eripuerunt.*

III

GRAMMARIAN

Distinguished physicians have often sought and found honour in fields far remote from the guild, and in literature, and more particularly in science, many have become famous, not a few while still active in practice. On our roll we find few who have sought relief in the, to many of us, arid fields of philology. The only one I recall in modern days is Robert Latham who was better known as a philologist than as a physician. So far as we know, Linacre never gave up the pursuit of medicine as a calling, but all through his life the infection of his early studies remained, and in hours of leisure he prepared two works which carried his fame as a grammarian into regions to which the name of the English physician had never penetrated, and justified Fuller's comment, " It is questionable whether he was a better Grammarian or Physician." Fed to inanition on the dry husks of grammar and with bitter school-boy memories of *Farrar on the Greek verb*, I can never pick up a text-book on the subject without a regret that the quickening spirit of Greece and Rome should have been for generations killed by the letter with which alone these works are concerned. It has been a great comfort to know that neither " Pindar nor Aeschylus had the faintest conception of these matters and that neither knew what was meant by an adverb or preposition or the rules of the moods and tenses" (Gomperz). And to find out who invented parts of speech and to be able to curse Protagoras by his Gods has been a source of inexpressible relief. But even with these feelings of hostility I find it impossible to pick up this larger work of Linacre without the thrill that stirs one at the recognition of successful effort—of years of persistent application. No teacher had had such distinguished pupils—Prince Arthur, the Princess Mary, Sir Thomas More, and Erasmus, the greatest scholar of the age. To Prince Arthur he dedicated his first work, Proclus *de Sphera.* Some years later, when tutor to the Princess Mary, he published two elementary grammars both in English. Of one of these, *Linacri Progymnasmata Grammatices Vulgaria* (no date), a unique copy is in the British Museum. There are verses by Linacre, by Sir Thomas More and by William Lily (Plate IX). Linacre's verses are addressed to the teachers and the boys. As Payne remarks, " Lily's verses refer to a former edition of the work, published under a false name and much corrupted, but now

restored to its pristine purity, and published
with the author's name. This is evidently the
lost grammar prepared by Linacre for St Paul's
school, but rejected by Colet" (see *Erasmi
Epistolae*, ed. Basel 1521, p. 420). The story
of the misunderstanding between the two scholars
is given in Knight's *Life of Colet* (pp. 135—139)
and the kind offices of Erasmus who urged
Colet not to believe all he heard of Linacre nor
irritate the scar (neque refricare eam cicatricem).
The second Latin Grammar has a more
important history. It is called *Rudimenta
Grammatices, Thomæ Linacri diligenter casti-
gata denuo, Londini in Aedibus Pynsonianis*,
4to, no date (Plate X). It is dedicated to the
Princess Mary of whose health as well as of
whose education he says he has the care.
A comparison of the two shows that the latter is
somewhat fuller, but it has the same arrange-
ment. There are epigrams by Richard Hirt

and William Lily. These smaller grammars of
Linacre had no vogue in England; but across
the channel in at least two generations French
boys were taught from it as Dame Quickly says
"to hick and to hack...and to call horum."
Falling into the hands of George Buchanan,
the poet-historian, it was translated by him for
the use of his pupil, Gilbert Kennedy, and
published in 1533 by Robert Etienne. Many
editions appeared on the continent, particularly
in France, where it was a favourite school book
for half a century, being reprinted as late as
1559. Were it not for the specific relation of
Montaigne how he was taught Latin in the
rational way one might have pictured the future
essayist seated at the feet of his tutor, the Scotch
exile, conning the *Rudimenta Grammatices*.

But Linacre's fame and reputation as a
grammarian rest on a much more important
work—the *de Emendata Structura Latini*

Sermonis, published in 1524, two months after the author's death (Plate XI). It is to be hoped that Pynson the publisher was able to show an early copy of this handsome quarto, as over few books has an author laboured for a longer period of time. It is touching to think that through all the busy period of his court employment and while the popular physician of the distinguished men of the country Linacre must have stolen a few hours each day for this work. There is but little doubt that to him and to it Erasmus refers in his well known description in the *Praise of Folly*. "I knew an old Sophister that was a Grecian, a Latinist, a mathematician, a philosopher, a physician, and all to the greatest perfection, who after three score years of experience in the world had spent the last twenty of them only in drudging to conquer the criticisms of grammar, and made it the chief parts of his prayers that his life might be so long spared till he had learned how rightly to distinguish betwixt the eight parts of speech, which no grammarian whether Greek or Latin had yet accurately done."

Linacre may well be the old grammarian of the well-known poem of Browning who doubtless got the idea from Erasmus. Two of the verses are worth quoting :

> "Back to his book then ; deeper drooped his head ;
>   Calculus racked him.
> Leaden before, his eyes grew dross of lead :
>   Tussis attacked him.
> 'Now, master, take a little rest,—not he !'
>   Not a whit troubled
> Back to his studies fresher than at first,
>   Fierce as a dragon.
> So with the throttling hands of Death at strife,
>   Ground he at grammar :
> Still, through the rattle, parts of speech were rife
>   While he could stammer.
> He settled Hoti's business—let it be !
>   Properly based Oun,
> Gave us the doctrine of the enclitic De,
>   Dead from the waist down."

Linacre, you remember, died of calculus or stone of the bladder.

Hallam's criticism of the work may be quoted: "This treatise is chiefly a series of Grammatical remarks relating to distinctions in the Latin language now generally known. It must have been highly valuable, and produced a considerable effect in England, where nothing of that superior criticism had been attempted. In order to judge of its proper merit, it should be compared with the antecedent works of Valla and Perotti. Every rule is supported by authorities; and Linacre, I observe, is far more cautious than Valla in asserting what is not good Latin, contenting himself for the most part with showing what is. It has been remarked that though Linacre formed his own style on the model of Quintilian, he took most of his authorities from Cicero. This treatise, the first-fruits of English erudition, was well received, and frequently printed on the Continent." The work never reappeared in

England, but it became very popular across the channel and was frequently reprinted, two of the editions are by distinguished scholars. It was issued in Paris by Stephanus in 1527, and a separate index in 1529. It was reprinted in Paris in 1532, 1540, 1543 and 1550. Camerarius of Bamberg issued an edition in 1538 (Leipzig), and in the letter of dedication to Lord Albert Margrave of Brandenburg, he dwells upon the importance of the grammatical art in the construction of discourse and for the study of pure, eloquent, copious and elegant speech. Philip Melanchthon edited an edition in 1531 for his little friend, Wilhelm Reiffenstein. The first few paragraphs of the introduction may be quoted as giving the impression made by the work on a distinguished scholar: "Here is offered a book of a most learned man, Linacre, on the syntax of the Latin language, which, as soon as I had perused it eagerly, I judged

would be of great service to students in learning
to speak Latin purely and aright and to form a
correct judging of the phrasing and all the
figures of the Latin language. For not only
does he hand down the usual rules, which,
though necessary to boys, are still by no means
sufficient for understanding the nature of the
language ; but he has also gone beyond prece-
dent and collected dissimilar examples in which
the varied construction of the same words
is discerned. And with singular prudence he
shows in the dissimilar construction of the
same words the diversity of meaning which
often deceives the unwary. He has examined
with wonderful diligence the force of co-predi-
cates whose great importance in varying the
meaning of other words is readily perceived by
men of intelligence. And so to me indeed no
more perfect writing of this character seems to
be extant."

Alas! for the poor little Swiss boy, for whom one cannot but feel sorry, as his friend was ambitious that he should go forth from school a perfected grammarian, an architect, an absolute artificer of language. He acknowledges that Linacre perhaps shows more assiduity than is needful in minutiae, but this is a subtilty which is demanded of a grammarian. What he praises particularly are the carefully chosen illustrations from the best authors. He rather qualifies his praise in one place by the remarkable statement that "the labour is in a mean subject, but the glory of a perfect grammarian is not mean." Forgotten to a great extent in England, Linacre's work as a grammarian held its own for two generations on the Continent, and an edition appeared as late as 1591. Milton refers to it in 1669 as " though very learned thought not fit to be read in schools " (Payne).

IV

THE LINACRE FOUNDATIONS

Linacre knew well the flourishing North Italian Universities,—Padua, where he graduated, Bologna and Ferrara and Pavia, and he was familiar with the organization through which they had achieved their great popularity. He had seen their flourishing medical schools, the resorts of students from all Europe, some of them in towns not so large as Oxford or Cambridge. He had found well arranged faculties with numerous lecturers, some of whom were highly paid. At Pavia in 1467 there were thirty-five teachers in the Medical Faculty and at Padua quite as many. For some years before his death, proposed benefactions for the study of medicine were discussed, and the University of Oxford having heard of them addressed to him two remarkable letters which are given in full by Johnson. Part of one is worth quoting as indicating a spirit of liberal friendliness towards science and medicine: "For how can you deserve better of our commonwealth, or by what memorial can you more honourably dedicate your name to the last remembrance of mankind, than in favouring and promoting the liberal arts, which, without the support and industry of the learned, would doubtless be exposed to destruction, or daily held in less esteem, a point on which your sober gravity and erudite judgment, by exciting the diligence of competent readers, will not confer less advantage, than will your bounteous generosity abundantly supply the means. Nay, of these the wise suggestions of your own judgment furnish the best proof, since you have chosen the science most subservient of all others to the necessities of humanity. For who even of the most potent has suitably requited the physician? The life we take from God, we retake from him: to his care we owe the preservation of the gift of existence, which we have received from the great creator of all things, and the restoration of it when in a state of decay. Hence we have not with Homer accounted the physician as a price for the many, but have enrolled him among mortals as a terrestrial deity. But why have we magnified the pre-eminence of the healing art to you, to whom all that relates to the excellence of this faculty is so entirely known?"

"The Lady Margaret," whose glorious monument is your college, had already established her Divinity professorships, but with these exceptions Linacre's bequests are memorable as the first attempts to endow University teaching. Centuries had to pass before the fulfilment of the wish which his practical mind had in this way indicated. Meanwhile through the centuries the collegiate tail continued to wag the University dog, and to this day in Oxford at least the higher faculties remain to a great extent unorganised and under the control of the Masters of Arts. The system has worked well for the squire but badly for learning, admirably for the schoolmaster and the parson, but badly for the nation since it permitted the old Universities to sleep on for years after science had cried her message from the house tops—awake! awake! for the light has come!

The foundations were made in Linacre's lifetime, but the *Diploma Regium*, dated the 12th of October, 1524, was issued only eight days before his death. Provision was made for two lectureships at Oxford and one at Cambridge, "dutifully his respect to his mother, double above his aunt," as Fuller says. There is nothing upon which to base the statement that Linacre had affiliations of any kind with Cambridge. Caius makes it, but there is no other reference. No doubt it was simply the act of a wise old man to encourage the study and teaching of medicine. It is interesting that here the deed of foundation was directly to the college; at Oxford to trustees. The deed was dated the 19th day of August in the 16th year of Henry the VIII, i.e., 1524, and the indenture was between " Thomas Lynacre doctor physicke and physicion to our Lord the Kyng Culbert by the suffraunce of God Bysshop of London Sir Thomas More Knyghte under Treasourer of England Maister John Stokesley clerk doctor of Divinite and William Shelley Serjaunt att Lawe and recorder of London on that oon partie. And Nicholas Metcalfe Clerke Maister of the College of Saint John the Evangeliste in Cambridge and the Fellowes

and Scolars of the same college on that other
partie." The " Belle and Lanthorne," Adlying
St in the parish of St Bennet, and £209 in gold
were given to the college, for which they were
to pay £12 a year for "a certayn lecture of
physicke to be founded and established in the
Universite of Cambridge." Every fourth year
the lecturer was to cease his " Redying" for the
space of half a year and he was to get only £6.
Nothing is said in the original deed as to the
subject of the lecture. By the Statutes of
Elizabeth, 1580, more precise directions are
given—the lecturer was to be a Master of Arts
at least, well versed in the works of Aristotle
and somewhat also on those books of Galen,
which Linacre had translated into Latin. The
office was continued in the Statutes of Victoria,
1849. The lecturer was to deliver courses on
Foods and Drugs, on the Care of Health, on
Methods of Healing, on Forensic Medicine or

on one or other of these subjects to be approved
by the Master. The college records have no
statement how the money grant was invested.
The property, " 17 Addle Hill," was purchased
by the Metropolitan Board of Works in 1865
for £4185.

The Linacre lecturers, for a list of whom I
am indebted to Mr Scott the Bursar and to
Dr Shore, illustrate the ups and downs of an
academic post. A majority of the men come
in that great group of the silent ones, the
voiceless, mere vowels and consonants to us,
without associations or traditions, and who are
to-day as though they had never been. Sixteen
of them have reached the distinction of the
Dictionary of National Biography. Among
these Baronsdale, Gisborne and Sir Thomas
Watson became Presidents of the Royal College
of Physicians. Collins, Pennington, Haviland
and Sir George Paget were Regius professors

of Physic. Paman (1670) was a Gresham Professor and a warm friend of Sydenham. The Edward Stillingfleet appointed in 1691 was not the well-known Bishop of Worcester, as is sometimes stated, but his son, who was Gresham Professor of Physic and afterwards took orders.

The two most interesting names are William Heberden and Thomas Watson. Of Heberden, the English Celsus, who was Linacre lecturer from 1734 to 1738, one could truly use the hyperbolean phrases of the Rusticus Placentinus of Padua in the 16th century—*Inter doctos doctissimus, inter doctissimos excellentissimus, inter excellentissimos eminentissimus.* Though in Latin his commentaries remain an English classic. Thomas Watson, afterwards Sir Thomas, the lecturer for 1822—26, was one of the most cultivated of the physicians of the 19th century, whose text-book on medicine, the delight of our fathers, is still worth reading for the style and for the admirable clinical description of disease. It was not always possible to find a Fellow of the college with medical qualifications. Twice only and that of late years has the college gone outside its own body—in the case of Sir George Paget and Dr Bradbury, the present distinguished Downing Professor of Physic who held the lectureship from 1872 to 1894. No injunction existed, as at Oxford, to go outside the college when a faculty Fellow was not available, and rather than allow the lectureship to lapse a non-medical Fellow was appointed. For example, Henry Briggs, 1592, was a distinguished mathematician, afterwards Savillian Professor of Astronomy at Oxford, and George Ashly, afterwards Master of the college, was an antiquary. Liberal souls, the Masters and Fellows of St John's have always encouraged the devotion of a Fellow to the muses, if needs be taking it for granted that he came

under the protection of Minerva Medica.   This
accounts for the otherwise apparent anomaly
that three distinguished Johnian poets have
been Linacre lecturers.   Robert Allott, elected
in 1604, was probably the editor of *England's
Parnassus* and the author of a number of minor
poems of whom I can find nothing to add to
what is given by Bullen in the *Dictionary of
National Biography* (1885).   In 1642 appears
the name of John Clieveland, the Cavalier poet,
who held the lectureship for only two years.
The *Dictionary of National Biography* states
that after holding a fellowship for six years he
had to make the choice of law or physic ;
nothing daunted, he took both and was admitted
to the physic line on January 31st 1642.   This
means, I suppose, that in order to keep him he
was attached to the Linacre foundation.   Let
us not begrudge him the emoluments if, as a
writer says (quoted in *Dictionary of National*

Biography) "he was the delight and ornament of St John's Society. What service as well as reputation he did it, let his orations and epistles speak ; to which the library oweth much of its learning, the chapel much of its pious decency and the college much of its renown." Fuller calls him "A general artist, pure Latinist, exquisite orator and (which was his masterpiece) eminent Poet," and adds that such "who have Clevlandized, endeavouring to imitate his Masculine Stile could never go beyond the Hermaphrodite, still betraying the weaker sex in their deficient conceits." Among your distinguished poets Mat. Prior holds, I trust, a treasured memory, if not with the Dons at any rate with the undergraduates, to whose lighter fancies and gay moods this 18th century Calverley should appeal. It was a great surprise to find his name in the list of Linacre lecturers. Appointed at a time when there

were cobwebs in his pocket, here too we may
forgive the Masters and Fellows of 1706 for
appointing the distinguished diplomat and poet
whose sole qualification for the position (as we
look at it, doubtless at that time the considera-
tions were personal) is the mirth and conse-
quently health-giving character of his poems.
In the distinguished man with whom has closed
the long list of Linacre lecturers were focussed
many of the most striking characteristics of his
predecessors, lay and medical. I doubt if
among the fifty there was one whose work he
could not have undertaken with a light heart.
We in the profession know him as a skilful and
learned physician. You are smarting under
the loss of a gifted colleague, but the public
fully realized that such high mental voltage
demanded a wider scope and this has been
found in the responsible position entrusted to
him by the Crown. Of few men in the pro-

fession since the days of the courtly Scarborough can it be more truly said

> Inter medicos Hippocrates,
> Inter mathematicos Euclides.

At Oxford the fate of Linacre's foundation has been less happy, the least happy indeed of the five distinct attempts made to further medical studies in Oxford. Nothing illustrates more glaringly the calamitous absence of faculty organization than the history of the Linacre, Tomlinson, Aldrichian, Lees and Litchfield bequests for Anatomy and Clinical Medicine at that university. We have seen that the Cambridge bequest took the form of a deed directly to this college; but at Oxford to four trustees, Sir Thomas More, Cuthbert Tunstall (at the time Bishop of London), John Stokesley and John Shelley were handed over the manors of Frognal and Tracies in the county of Kent, by letters patent dated the 12th of October,

4—2

1524. The lands were assigned to the Wardens
and Freemen of the Mercers' Company who
were to hand over the sum of £30 sterling
annually for the support and maintenance of
the lectures. It is not quite clear from the deed
of trust what was to be the relation of the
trustees to the Mercers' Company, and the
Warden of Merton tells me that at present
there is no connection of the Manors with the
Mercers' Company. As Johnson states, the
choice of trustees was singularly unfortunate,
though all were personal friends of the bene-
factor. More was deeply involved in affairs
of State, Tunstall engrossed in business of the
sees, Stokesley was heresy hunting, and John
Shelley, who was no doubt the business member
of the trustees, had "neither the influence nor
power to execute the provisions of the licence."
It was not until the third year of Edward VI,
1550, that the Oxford lectureships were estab-

lished, not as independent foundations but in connection with Merton College. It was most natural that Tunstall, the surviving trustee, should have asked this college to take charge of the trust. The affairs in the University were very unsettled. There was indeed a Professor of Medicine, but there was no faculty of Medicine, and for more than two centuries Merton enjoyed the reputation of the most distinguished medical college in England. Roger Bacon, who wrote extensively on medicine, was a Merton man, and the most famous English physician of the 13th century, John of Gaddesden, taught medicine at Merton. The *Rosa Anglica* (beautiful manuscripts of which are in the college library) was one of the first medical books printed by an Englishman. (Pavia, 1492.) John Chambers, a friend and contemporary of Linacre, a fellow founder with him of the College of Physicians, was Warden of the college, and a little later John Clement, a Fellow of Merton, afterwards became President of the College of Physicians.

A higher and lower lectureship was instituted, the former to be held for life, the latter to be for three years.   The readers were to lecture on Hippocrates and Galen.   Robert Barnes or Barons was made the first "higher lecturer," George James, the first "lower lecturer," was appointed in 1559.   Through the kindness of the Warden I have had a list of the lecturers. There is only too much truth in what B. W. Henderson says in his history of the college : " The happy inheritor of the Linacre bequest received his money gladly and made no pretence of work, although to save appearances and salve consciences it was almost invariably the case that the Fellow elected at Merton to the sinecure was also Doctor of Medicine." Only a few men of distinction have held the lectureship. Roger Gifford was a man of note in the 16th century and after a somewhat stormy life at the college during the struggles between the Catholics and Protestants he went to London and became physician to Queen Elizabeth and President of the College of Physicians. Many fine volumes from his library are among the treasures at Merton. He was the lower lecturer in 1561—62. John Chamber, appointed lower lecturer in 1579, is still remembered at Merton by the two Chamber Post-Masterships awarded to candidates from Eton.

Theodore Gulston, elected to the lower lectureship in 1609, had an interesting career and is remembered to-day by the Gulstonian lectures delivered annually at the Royal College of Physicians. Many of his fine folios are in the library of Merton College.

Edward Lapworth, lower lecturer, 1619, was

a scholarly physician with a taste for poetry.
He was appointed the first Sedleian reader in
natural philosophy. There is a good account
of him in the *Dictionary of National Biography*. Daniel Whistler, the higher lecturer
appointed for three years, 1647—1650, had a
distinguished career and became President of
the Royal College of Physicians in 1683. He
has a place in medical literature as the author
of the first published work on Rickets (In-
augural thesis at Leyden, 1645, *De Morbo
Puerili Anglorum*) for which he proposed the
name of *Paedossplanchnosteocaces*. He was also
Gresham Professor of Geometry. Edmund
Dickinson, the higher lecturer, 1653—1669,
was for many years a practitioner in Oxford and
afterwards a well-known physician in London.
He established a philosophy the principles of
which were a mixture of the Pentateuch, the
atomic theory, and the Greek and Roman

writers. On his monument in the church of St Martin's in the Fields is a laudatory inscription in which occurs the lines :—

> Et, quod raro, Medicus stabilivit Theologum
> Theologus Medicum.

William Coward, appointed in 1685, achieved distinction by having his theological and philosophical books burnt by the common hangman at the command of the House of Commons. Gilbert Trowe or Trewe, appointed first in 1715, appears to have held sometimes the higher, sometimes the lower lectureship with a few interruptions until 1753. He became Professor of Botany in 1724. A Dr Ruding held one of the lectureships with a few intervals from 1747 to 1789. Samuel Kilmer, who did good work for Merton in collecting the Archives of the College, was appointed lower in 1746, higher in 1789, and then held both together until the year 1815. As a result of the

University commission in 1854 the Professorship of Physiology was founded and attached to
Merton and called the Linacre Professorship
with a stipend of £800 a year. In May, 1860,
George Rolleston, M.D., was elected Professor
and with him begins the new era of Anatomical
and Physiological studies in Oxford, and under
the auspices of Sir Henry Acland the Medical
School has gradually revived. In 1882 the
Linacre chair was changed to that of Compara-
tive Anatomy and has been held by Mosley,
1882, Ray Lankester, 1891, Weldon, 1899, and
Bourne, 1906.

Linacre's name is indissolubly associated
with a much more important foundation—the
College of Physicians of London of which he
was one of the founders and the first president,
in the year 1518. At this period the license to
practice was in the hands of the church, in fact
it can scarcely be said that medicine existed

as a distinct profession. There were a few physicians who were often ecclesiastics, a few surgeons, and the general practice was done by barber surgeons and apothecaries. The charter granted to the College allowed it to regulate the practice of physic in London and for seven miles around. Four years later the privileges of the College were extended over the whole of England. Only graduates of Oxford and Cambridge were allowed to practice without a license. But it was many years before the bishops gave up their rights, and a remnant of this ecclesiastical privilege persists in the power of the Archbishop of Canterbury to confer the doctorate—the Lambeth degree. Linacre took a very active interest in the affairs of the College which at first met in his house on Knight-Rider St, the site of which is still in the possession of the College. His library, which he also left to the College, was burned at the great fire; but he left what has been much more valuable to English medicine,—an example of a life of devotion to learning, to medicine and to the interests of humanity.

The history of the two pictures of Linacre, which are here shown, is of interest. The original of the first (Frontispiece), the more familiar one so often reproduced, is at Windsor, and good copies are in the College of Physicians and in All Souls College. Doubts as to its authenticity have been expressed. Mr Lionel Cust writes : " The portrait bears the brand C.P. on the back, which shows that it belonged to Charles I when Prince of Wales. It does not however appear in Vander Doort's catalogue in 1639, though it appears in that of James II's pictures in 1688 as No. 527, 'An old man's head with a letter in his hand, by Holbein.' In the catalogue of the pictures at Kensington Palace in 1818 it is entered as No.

182, ' Portrait of the celebrated Linacre founder of the College of Physicians...P. C. Quintin Matsys.' It is not certain when the name of Linacre got attached to the portrait. The man represented in the portrait holds a letter on which is the date 1527. Linacre died October 24th, 1524 and it does not happen that he left England during the last twenty five years of his life....Unfortunately the portrait has been subsequently accepted as the true portrait of the famous founder of the College of Physicians in London, a contention which it would be difficult to establish." It is suggested that the date on the paper of the Windsor portrait, 1527, is a mistake for 1521, which appears to be the figures on the College of Physicians copy. It is stated that this copy was made as late as 1810, but both Sir William Armstrong and Mr Lionel Cust are of the opinion that it is very much older, indeed, by an old master. Mr

William Fleming of the College of Physicians, who has paid much attention to its history and has been kind enough to give me much information about Linacre, has found the following reference: "Quintin Matsys too painted Aegidius with which Sir Thomas More was so pleased that he wrote a panegyric on the painter. Aegidius held a letter in his hand from Sir Thomas with his hand writing so well imitated that More could not distinguish it himself. Quintin too in the year 1521 drew the picture of the celebrated physician, Dr Linacre[1]." This suggests that after all the features which have been made so familiar to us by the frequent reproduction of this picture may in reality be those of the learned scholar and physician. The other picture which so well represents the old grammarian is from a

---

[1] *Anecdotes of Painting in England,* by Mr Horace Walpole, 1762, vol. I., p. 65.

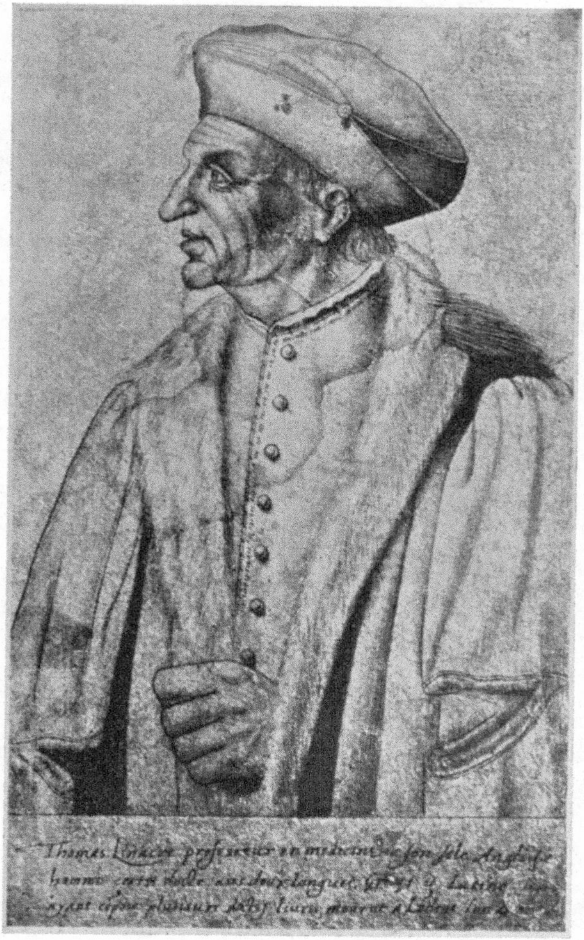

Plate II

Portrait of Linacre at the British Museum

sketch in the British Museum (Plate II). About it Mr Sidney Colvin kindly sent me the following note: "The drawing is by a French hand, of about A.D. 1600, evidently copied from a picture (which is not now known to exist). It shows a man with a shaved face deeply lined, a long drooping nose and parted lips, one half length in profile to the left, wearing a fur lined cloak and a doctor's cap, and has at foot this inscription—'Thomas Linacre Professor au medicine a son isle Anglaise, homme certes docte aux deux langues Grescq̃ et Latine, lequel ayant cõpase plusieurs doctes livres, mourut a Lõdres l'an de võre Seigr., 1524.'" The features in the two pictures are not very much alike. That of Quintin Matsys represents a man much younger looking than we can suppose Linacre to have been in 1521.

I cannot conclude without expressing my indebtedness to Johnson's *Life*, 1835, and to the articles on Linacre in the *Dictionary of National Biography* and in the reprint of the *de Temperamentis* by Dr J. F. Payne, the learned Harveian Librarian of the Royal College of Physicians.

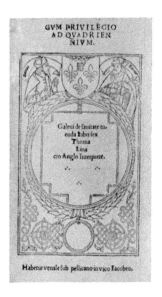

Symphonia Plato

nis cum Aristotele: & Galeni cū Hippocrate D. Symphoriani Chāpenj. Hippocratica philosophta eiusdem. Platonica medicina de duplici mundo: cum eiusdē scholijs. Speculum medicinale platonicum: & apologia literarū humaniorum.

Quæ omnia vēnundantur ab Iodoco Badio.

Plate III

Symphonia Platonis

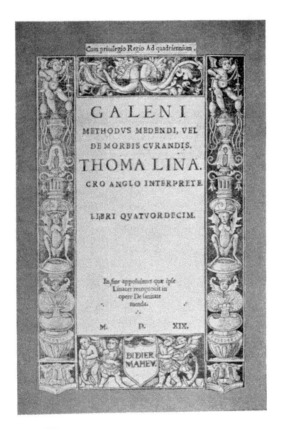

GVM PRIVILEGIO
AD QVADRIEN
NIVM.

Galeni de sanitate tu-
enda libri sex
Thoma
Lina
cro Anglo Interprete.

Habentur venale sub pellicano invico Iacobeo.

Plate IV

de Sanitate Tuenda

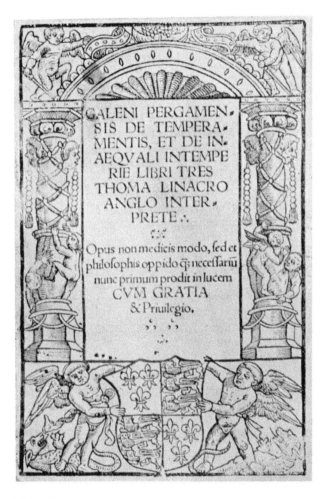

Plate V

Methodus Medendi

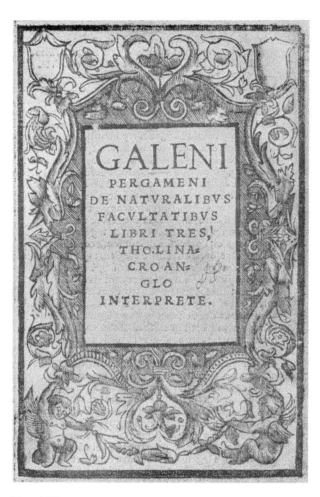

GALENI PERGAMEN-
SIS DE TEMPERA-
MENTIS, ET DE IN-
AEQVALI INTEMPE
RIE LIBRI TRES
THOMA LINACRO
ANGLO INTER-
PRETE ∴

Opus non medicis modo, fed et
philofophis oppido q̃ neceffariũ
nunc primum prodit in lucem
CVM GRATIA
& Priuilegio.

Plate VI

de Temperamentis

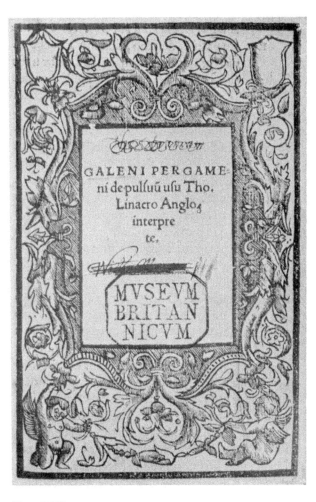

GALENI
PERGAMENI
DE NATVRALIBVS
FACVLTATIBVS
LIBRI TRES,
THO. LINA=
CRO AN=
GLO
INTERPRETE.

Plate VII

de Naturalibus Facultatibus

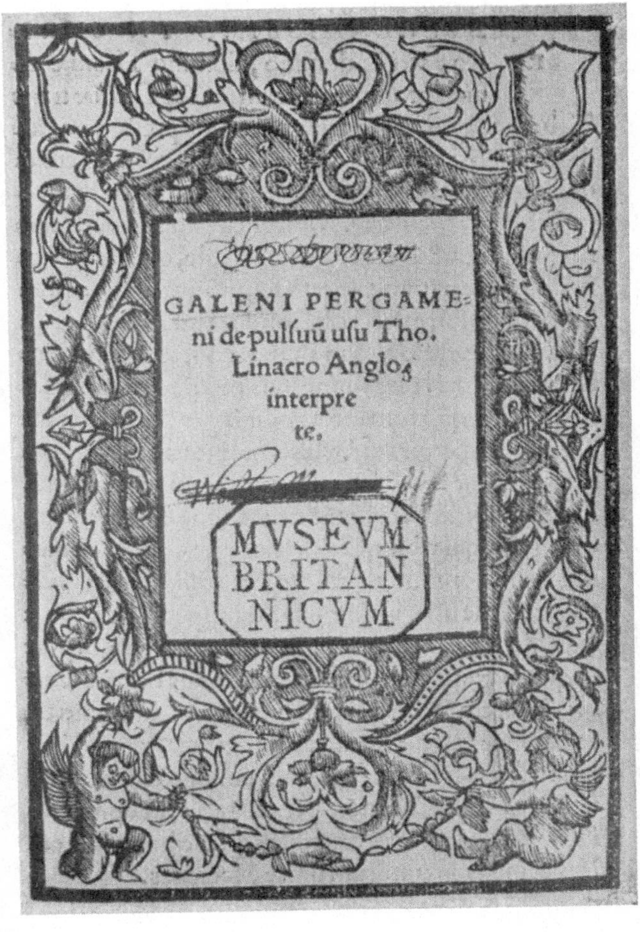

GALENI PERGAME=
ni de pulſuū uſu Tho.
Linacro Angloᵹ
interpre
te.

MVSEVM
BRITAN
NICVM

Plate VIII

de Pulsuum Usu

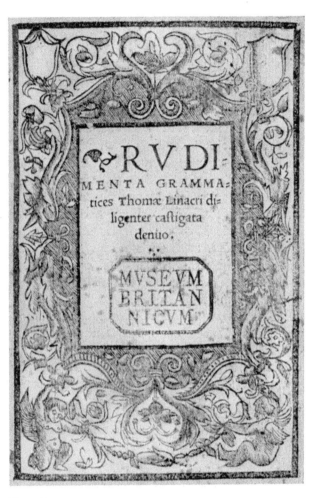

Linacri ad pceptores ptie & pueros
Pzimum hec que patria libuit conscribere lingua
    Haud quaæ inuitus plegito Angle puer
Nec tibi concisus videar si fozte quibusdam
    Ista legis missis que potui adstruere
Sic placitum est de te pzimu cepisse periclum
    Ad nozma explesse:an semi repleta queas
At tu pzeceptoz qui multa nouata notabis
    Quozum nec ratio hic sat sua costiterit:
Inde labozaris nolim.mox illa dabuntur
    Quis tibi plectis:fiet in hisce satis
Ergo vel ista cubans ambas securus in aures
    Interea pueros qualiacunæ doce.

Thome mozi in pgymnasmata linacri.

Qui leget hec sensim docti pzecepta linacri
    Dicere(si teneat que legit inde)volet
Post tot gramatices imensa volumina paruus
    Non tamen incassum pzodiit iste liber
Exiguus liber est.Sed gemme moze nitentis
    Exiguo magnum cozpoze fert pzecium.

Guliel. Lilij in pgymnasmata Gra-
matic.Linacri a plagiario vindicata

Pagina que falso latuit sub nomine nuper
    Que fuit et multo comaculata luto
Nunc tandem authozis pscribens nomina veri
    Linacri dulces pura recepit aquas

Plate IX

Progymnasmata Grammatices Vulgaria

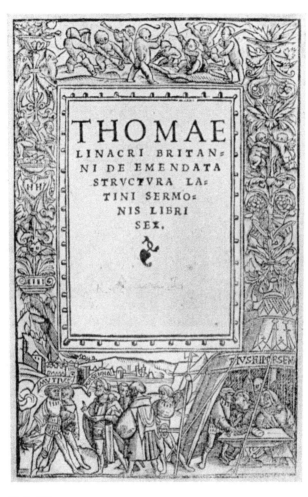

&❧RVDI-
MENTA GRAMMA=
tices Thomæ Linacri di=
ligenter caſtigata
denuo.

MVSEVM
BRITAN
NICVM

Plate X

Rudimenta Grammatices

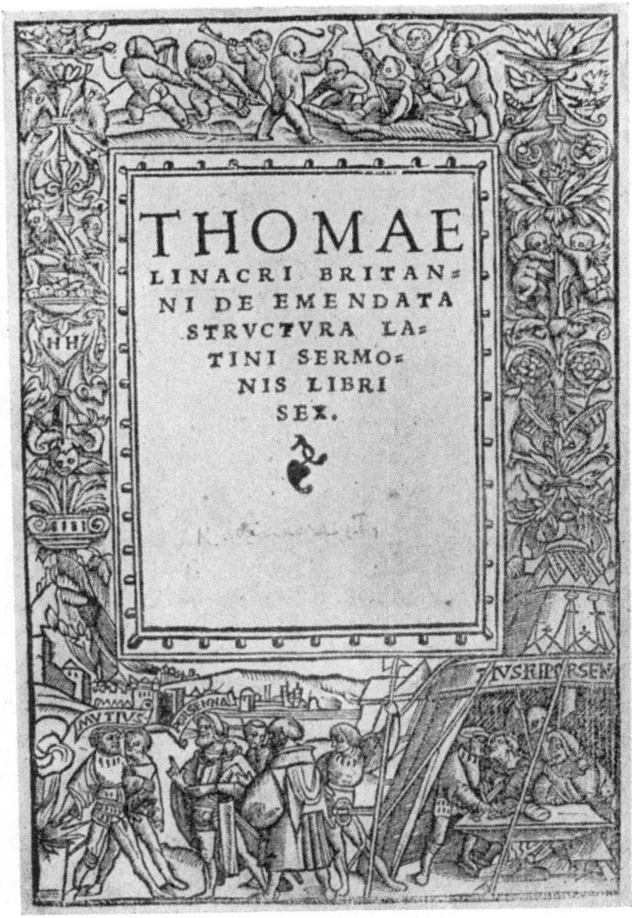

THOMAE

LINACRI BRITAN=
NI DE EMENDATA
STRVCTVRA LA=
TINI SERMO-
NIS LIBRI
SEX.

Plate XI

de Emendata Structura Latini Sermonis

Printed in the United States
By Bookmasters